What Makes Me Fat?

How to Eliminate Obesity Naturally!

By M. Usman

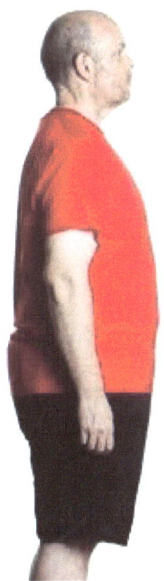
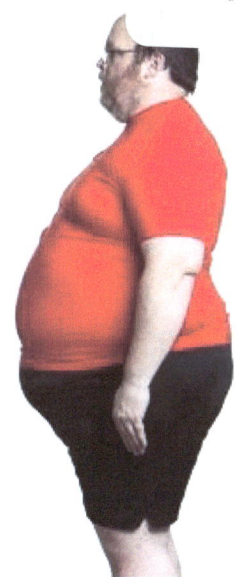

Health Learning Series

Mendon Cottage Books

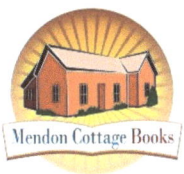

JD-Biz Publishing

Disclaimer

The information is this book is provided for informational purposes only. It is not intended to be used and medical advice or a substitute for proper medical treatment by a qualified health care provider. The information is believed to be accurate as presented based on research by the author.

The contents have not been evaluated by the U.S. Food and Drug Administration or any other Government or Health Organization and the contents in this book are not to be used to treat cure or prevent disease.

The author or publisher are not responsible for the use or safety of any diet, procedure or treatment mentioned in this book. The author or publisher is not responsible for errors or omissions that may exist.

Warning

The Book is for informational purposes only and before taking on any diet, treatment or medical procedure it is recommended to consult with your primary care provider.

Our books are available at

1. Amazon.com

2. Barnes and Noble

3. Itunes

4. Kobo

5. Smashwords

6. Google Play Books

Table of Contents

Introduction

"Overall, more than 10% of the world's population is obese"
(World Health Organization- WHO)

Superfluous food and the ease with which we can attain all the things we need has made physical activity almost extinct. It's safe to say that obesity is the gift of modern era; a gift that can potentially be deadly. For instance, according to the same report almost 2.8 million adults die each year of obesity! If you're suffering from this disease of modern era, this last point should give ample reason for you to try get rid of obesity. This book discusses how dangerous obesity can be and gives you a complete plan regarding how you can get rid of this curse of the modern era.

Is obesity as evil as it sounds? Yes, it is. Not only it makes you look unfit but also makes you susceptible to a number of health hazards like high blood pressure, metabolic disorders, diabetes, stroke, joint complications, cancer and heart attack.

It's ironic that how the hearts and souls of people tremble when they hear of diseases like cancer, heart attack and stroke. Obesity; who cares about it? I love food, I live for eating, and eating is my life. People try to hide this foe behind these statements. Why wait for a heart attack or a stroke? Why not try to nip the evil in its bud? I feel no hesitation in saying that obesity is the mother of hundreds of other diseases. It's not a disease in itself but is the risk factor of several other maladies.

By now you would be wondering; "if obesity is so dangerous then it should take a magical pill to get rid of it". That magical pill is in your hands. A healthy lifestyle is the only way to get rid of this condition. Who needs a doctor when you can cure a condition all by yourself? The major portion of this book focuses on describing the dietary habits, different exercise, herbal alternatives and home remedies to burn extra fat. But sometimes, things do get serious and you need a doctor. The last few pages describe the medicinal and surgical remedies of obesity.

SECTION ONE

What is obesity? - The story behind

What do you understand by the word "obesity"? Being obese doesn't simply mean that you've put on some extra weight. In medical terms, obesity is defined as the condition in which excess amount of fats starts accumulating in body tissues. These unwanted fats exert negative effects on body, leading to many health hazards.

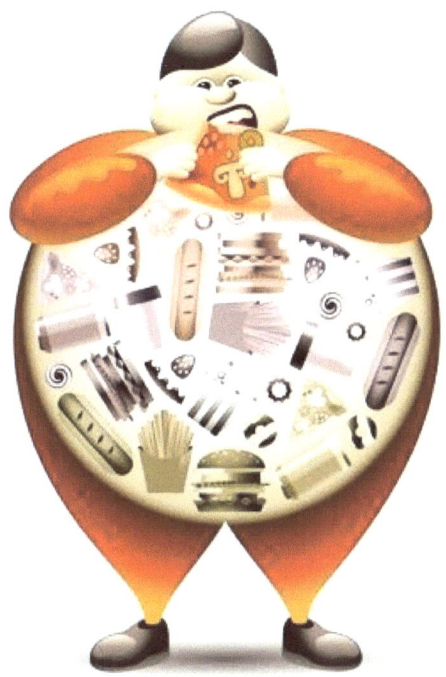

Obesity is a matter of concern because it poses many threats to health. Being overweight contributes to increase the risks of cardiovascular diseases, Type

2 diabetes, hypertension, hyperlipidemia, cancers, gynecological problems and strokes. Gaining weight is easy but to lose it is quite difficult. Treatment of obesity is inevitable for minimizing the risks of obesity linked diseases. But you can't expect to treat obesity with shortcuts. You'll have to be patient to obtain your desired results.

Body mass index (BMI):

BMI is a scale for statistical measurement of obesity. It's the ratio of body mass in kg to the square of height in meters. An adult person having BMI ranging from 25-29.9 is considered to be overweight. If your BMI is above 30, you're obese.

Causes of obesity - why am I getting fat?

High caloric foods:

The main culprit behind this prevailing health hazard is the food we consume. The foods you're eating are high in calorie. Consuming too much calories leads to weight gain. Your body can handle only a limited number of calories per day. If you eat calories more than your body needs, the extra calories will be converted to fats.

Sedentary life style:

Just have look at your lifestyle. You'll be able to see that how lazy and sedentary life we are living today. The invention of modern technologies and machines has made us too lazy. We spend our leisure time in watching TV shows, playing computer and mobile games. The concept of healthy physical activities was forgotten a long ago. Without indulging in some physical activity, you won't be able to burn the calories that you have consumed. A report published in American Journal Of Preventive medicine states:

"Children who have television in their rooms are much more likely to be obese or overweight"

The basis behind this report is that such children love to eat while watching television and TV reduces the level of physical activities to absolute zero.

Lack of sleep:

Lack of sleep is also responsible for weight gain. When you stay awake for a longer time, your hormones get disturbed. Imbalance in hormones increases your appetite and cravings for sugary foods.

Medical problems:

Some people gain weight for unknown reason. Obesity can be the outcome of various medical conditions like thyroid problems, Cushing syndrome and Polycystic ovarian syndrome (POS). In such cases, you can't stop gaining weight until you treat the underlying disease.

Genetic:

Your genes also play a role in causing obesity. If the origin of your obesity is genetic, it's very difficult to treat it.

Age and sex:

Females are more prone to get obese as compared to males and obesity usually progresses with age.

"Three Fs" are very common, doctors say. Female, Forty, and Fat.

SECTION TWO

Foods you should eat to lose weight –

"Eat healthy, to stay healthy"

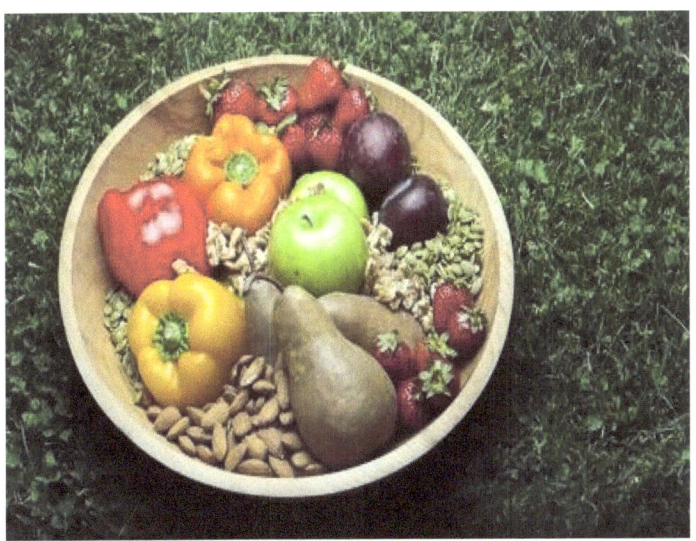

Oats:

If you want to lose weight then first thing you must try is adding oats and whole grains to your diet. Oats are enriched with fibers and proteins. High fiber content of oats makes you feel full for longer time as compared to other foods. Having a bowl of oatmeal in breakfast daily might help you lose weight. Oats maintain the sugar level in blood because they contain complex carbohydrates/sugars which are released slowly into the blood.

Green tea :

How can the significance of green tea be forgotten in promoting weight loss? 2-3 cups of green tea daily are good for losing weight. Green tea contains "polyphenols" which help in digesting triaclyglycerides (fats) stored in body. It also contains anti oxidants called "epigalletocatechin gallate" which boosts the body metabolism. Burn more and more fats by drinking green tea to get a slim and smart figure.

Olive oil

Have you ever given it a thought that whether the oils you use for cooking are safe or not? Now, it's time to open your eyes and face the reality. You need to know that most of the cooking oils are not good for health as they contain cholesterol and unhealthy or bad fats (saturated fats). These fats deposit in body tissues and make us fat. Not only this, bad fats increase the chances of heart diseases as well. But it's never too late to make a change. Olive oil is the best replacement of these hazardous cooking oils. Olive oil contains very strong anti oxidants known as omega 3 fatty acids which speed up the metabolism of bad fats.

Mushrooms:

Apart from being delicious, mushroom is the best food for people who want to lose weight. Mushrooms are a good source of proteins. These are a perfect replacement of red meat. Try to eat mushrooms instead of eating fatty red meat to get more flavor and nutrition without getting obese.

Avocados:

Avocado contains fats yet there is no need to get afraid because avocados are full of healthy fats. It might intrigue you that how can healthy fats promote fat loss? Here is your answer: avocados are enriched with monounsaturated fats (MUFA's) which keep your lipid profile in balance. These fatty acids are easily metabolized by body. Unlike bad fats, these healthy fats don't have the tendency to stay for longer time in tissues. If you want to melt away the stubborn belly fat then eat avocados and see the prominent result.

Beans:

If you're asked about the richest source of protein, the first thing that comes in your mind is meat. Yes, meat is the excellent source of proteins but the meat we consume also contains saturated fats which are not good for health. But meat is not the only source of essential proteins because you've got many other foods which can fulfill your protein requirements. One such food is beans. Beans serve the same purpose as meat. You can cut down your meat intake by adding beans in your diet. Beans have got high nutritional value due to their high fiber content. Fibers give your food a bulk which helps to satisfy your hunger. Fibers also regulate your digestive system and body metabolism.

The reason for supporting beans as the best choice for weight loss is their low glycemic index. If you are looking for a low carbohydrate diet as a solution for obesity, beans are certainly good option. Beans contain complex carbohydrates which maintain the blood sugar level and suppress the insulin release, which may promote weight loss.

Berries:

Do you know that blueberries and blackberries contain up to 85% water? This interesting fact seems to be responsible for their role in accelerating weight loss. Juicy nature of berries makes them a perfect food for losing weight. Eating a handful of berries will satisfy your hunger quickly. Berries also contain antioxidants and soluble fibers which aid in weight loss. Obese people are more prone to heart diseases because the cholesterol level is usually high in their bodies. Soluble fiber present in berries lowers the cholesterol level by binding with it and eliminating it from body. The healthy anti oxidants, on the other hand, boosts up the metabolism of bad fats.

Salmon:

Salmon fish is the healthiest food as it contains a great combination of lean proteins, low calories and mono unsaturated fats (MUFA's). Salmon is rich is omega 3 fatty acids which play an indirect role in weight loss. They lower the LDL (low density lipoprotein) or bad cholesterol in body and reduce the risks of heart diseases in fat people. Omega 3 fatty acids have the anti oxidant abilities. Antioxidants are necessary for hastening the fat burning process. When the stored fats are oxidized or burned, the oxygen free radicals and toxins are produced which enter into fat cells, damage their structure and hinder the burning of fats. Anti oxidants combat these free radicals and speed up the fat metabolism.

Apples:

Apples is the another superb food with low calories, high fiber and a lot of vitamins and minerals. An apple contains about 5 grams of fibers. Eating 3 apples a day will provide you with 15 grams of fibers. Fibers will distend your stomach and you'll feel satisfied for longer. The best way to lose weight is to eat an apple either before the meals or between the meals as it will fill you up and you won't be able to eat much.

There are still some other ways through which apples promote fat loss. Apples contain "pectin", a soluble dietary fiber, which binds with glucose and limit its absorption through intestine. These fibers also benefit you by lowering cholesterol in body. The vitamins and minerals in apples fortify the overall metabolism which enables your body to burn more calories and fats. All these health benefits of apples contribute to visible weight loss.

As the saying goes:

"An apple a day, keeps the doctor away"

Cabbage Soup:

The bitter taste of cabbage may offend you but believe it or not, cabbage soup diet is the fastest way to lose weight. Consuming a bowl of cabbage soup daily for one week will help you lose up to 10 pounds of weight. Cabbage soup contains low proteins, low carbohydrates, high fiber and less vitamins and minerals. Thus, by exhausting the energy reserves of body the cabbage soup stimulates the burning of more and more calories to compensate for energy loss. But remember, you shouldn't continue this diet plan for more than a week.

Eat veggies; Your best buddies!!

Lean meat:

Including lean meat in your diet plan is effective in driving weight lose because it contains small amount fats and low calories. Lean meat is entirely composed of essential proteins which are necessary for building up your muscle mass. By building up more muscle mass you are actually increasing your basal metabolic rate. The higher the metabolic rate, the more will be the calorie burning and slightest will be the chance of gaining weight.

Brown rice:

Brown rice is the unrefined form of white rice. Brown rice is enriched with a lot of nutrients like magnesium, selenium and vitamin B complex. For all those dieters who are looking for low calorie and high fiber diet, brown rice is among those foods which fulfill these criteria. Brown rice is preferred over white rice because they're whole grains which white rice is not. Brown rice contains a lot of starches or complex carbohydrates as compared to white rice. These complex carbohydrates break down slowly and release glucose gradually which prevents the sudden spike in insulin level. Insulin is regarded as the fat storing hormone. After the utilization of glucose by tissues, the insulin stores the spare glucose in the form of fat. Eating brown rice will help you a lot in losing weight by suppressing this insulin release. Now while dieting you can enjoy eating rice without consuming many calories.

Foods to avoid- "Think before you eat"

Fast foods:

Fast foods are the worst foods for your health. Avoid them as much as possible if you are interested in reducing your weight. Cooking oil used for preparing these junk foods is harmful for health. These things are not nutritious as they contain a huge number of calories, bad fats and carbohydrates.

Avoid sugary foods:

Sugary foods are actually the sweet poisons which kill you slowly. We always accuse fatty foods for making us obese. But you don't know that carbohydrate rich foods do more harm. Sugary foods disturb insulin level in blood. When you eat carbohydrate rich foods, the glucose level raises in blood. To bring it back to normal, insulin hormone is released. Insulin facilitates the utilization of glucose by muscle and other body tissues. The glucose that is spared is converted by insulin into fats, which are then stored in fat cells of body. The continuous consumption of sugary foods keeps your insulin level always high. A time comes when your tissues stop responding to insulin. Glucose becomes unable to enter the cells. This is known as "insulin resistance". The only option left for insulin is to covert more and more glucose into fats. Increased insulin resistance makes you prone to type 2 diabetes.

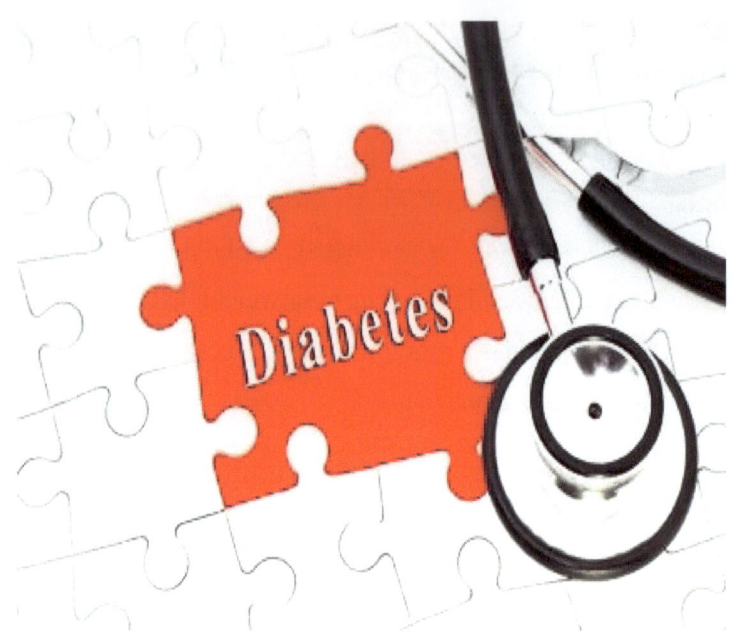

Milk products:

Milk is a good source of calcium, minerals and vitamins but it contains a high amount of saturated fats. These fats tend to deposit in body, which causes obesity. Avoiding milk products may help you lose some stored, unhealthy fats.

Baked products:

Chocolate cakes, pan cakes, cup cakes, muffins, pizzas seem to be very tempting and delicious. But this is your biggest mistake to eat these low nutritional value foods. They contain calories multiple times more than your average daily requirement. Satisfying your appetite with these high caloric foods will make you overweight and obese

Avoid beverages:

We are fond of colas, sodas and artificially made juices. It seems that our life is incomplete without them. These beverages have zero nutritional value. Drinking these cold drinks will load your body with a huge number of calories and sugar, leading you to put on weight.

Fried foods:

Fried foods like potato chips are your enemies if you are trying to get rid of obesity. Frying the foods adds extra calories to them. You may love to eat French fries but they will make you put on weight.

A quick check list:

Foods to eat	Foods to avoid
Vegetables like cabbage	Junk food
Fruits like avocados	Fizzy drinks and colas
Beans	Bakery products
Lean meat	Dairy products
Salmon fish	Ready to eat foods
Brown rice	Red meat.
Green Tea	White rice

Home remedies for weight loss - "Try them and don't regret"

Honey and lemon:

You might get confused that how honey will help you lose weight? Honey isn't like the table sugar we use. Honey in its raw form contains many nutrients like vitamins, minerals, amino acids, antioxidants. Honey has low glycemic index as compared to refined sugars which means that it doesn't disturb the blood sugar level. The anti oxidants in honey act as the boosters of body metabolism. They regulate the cholesterol level and stimulate the loss of unwanted fats.

Honey and lemon juice is a wonderful home remedy to fight against obesity. Add two tablespoon of honey and three table spoon of lime juice in a glass of lukewarm water. Mix it with a spoon and drink it. Having this honey and lemon juice mixture in the morning and evening is really helpful in melting away the stubborn fats.

Honey, the magic elixir, is being used for thousand of years. It's uses are written in the oldest greek and chinese manuscripts.

Drink water:

It's suggested to drink a glass of water for before taking a meal. Researchers say that those who drink a glass of water before every meal, they eat less. The reason behind this is very simple and logical. Drinking a glass of water before having meals cut down your appetite, therefore you tend to eat less.

Taking a glass of lukewarm in morning, empty stomach, will flush out the harmful toxins from body which might be responsible for your poor health and weight gain

Ginger:

Ginger has gained medicinal importance over the past few years due to its various health benefits. Ginger plays an interesting role in weight loss. Ginger promotes weight loss in following ways;

- When you eat ginger, it generates heat in the body which prompts burning of stored calories in body.
- Ginger has the properties to boost up the metabolic rate of body.
- Ginger elevates the serotonin level in blood, the hormone which suppresses hunger.
- You can lower your cholesterol level by chewing a fresh ginger daily.

There are many ways to use ginger as home remedy for weight loss. Add ½ teaspoon of ginger powder in a half glass of water and drink this mixture daily to cut down some extra pounds. Sipping ginger tea 2-3 time a day is another home remedy for obesity. Or you can mix 2 table spoon of ginger juice with 3 table spoon of honey. Having this mixture twice a day helps in losing weight.

Apple cider vinegar:

Apple cider vinegar is used as an effective home remedy for obesity. The following facts about vinegar make it a perfect choice for weight loss programs:

- Apple cider vinegar contains a lot of fibers called pectin. Pectin fibers from a gel like substance in stomach which expands it and makes you feel full and satisfied. This ultimately suppresses appetite.
- Consuming too much sodium cause the water retention in body, responsible for increasing the weight. Apple cider vinegar contains a high concentration of potassium which replaces sodium in body. By keeping the sodium low, the water retention is reduced and weight gain is prevented.
- Vinegar improves the metabolic rate. The higher metabolic rate means that more calories are being burned which causes weight loss.
- Apple cider vinegar not only aids in digestion process but it also limits the absorption of fats through intestine.

Mix two tea spoon of organic apple cider vinegar in a cup of water. Drink it up. Sip this mixture several times a day to lose a few pounds weight. You can also add a teaspoon of lemon juice in it to enhance the taste.

Avoid snacks between meals:
Many people have the habit of taking snacks when they feel hungry without being aware of the fact that these snacks can add more to the fat load in their body. Taking snacks like chips and biscuits in between the meals may be the cause behind your weight gain. You can't lose weight in an effective manner till you stop nibbling between meals. You'll have to manage your hunger if you really want to lose weight. The best way to avoid these snacks is to replace them with some fruits. Fruits won't affect your weight because they

contain nutritious vitamins and minerals that not only keep you active but also stimulate the weight loss

Frequent meals:

In daily routine, most of the people eat 2-3 meals per day. But if you want a real and promising solution for your extra weight, you must take frequent small meals a day rather than eating 2 large meals. It's advised to take 5-6 meals after the interval of every 2-3 hours. Consuming small meals benefits you by improving the metabolic rate. Obviously, when you eat in small amount, your body will be able to digest it rapidly and less calories will be absorbed. This means that more calories are being burned than are being absorbed, which accelerates the weight loss.

Carrot juice:

Drinking carrot juice is a good way to lose weight. Carrot juice is low in calories but rich in vitamin and minerals. Having a glass of carrot juice daily in the morning reduces your craving for meal.

Salads:

While making a weight loss program, the first thing you must do is add salads to your diet. Having a bowl of salad in noon, daily, will cut down your appetite and you will feel full and satisfied throughout the day. But bear that in your mind that the salads you are eating should not be laden with cream and mayonnaise dressings.

Peppers:

Add pepper and chillies to your meal because they have got thermogenic properties. Peppers produce heat in body and help in burning more calories. They also make your food to look colourful, tempting and delicious.

Walk after eating a meal:

Stop! if you are done with your meal and are now going to sleep. Look at your fat belly once. Don't you want to know how it got there? The culprit for your fat belly is lying down immediately after taking a meal. Perhaps, you have forgotten the importance of taking a walk after having a meal. Doing a brisk walk, 5-10 minutes after finishing your meal, for 15-20 minutes is an effective strategy to lose weight. Walking keeps you active and aids you in digesting food rapidly. While being active, you are utilizing more calories than being absorbed.

Eat homemade food:

Things have changed over the past few years. There were days when homemade foods were considered more nutritious, healthy and tasty. But unfortunately the eating habits have entirely changed in this modern era of civilization. So far we've succeeded in raising our living standards but at the cost of our precious health. Now you can see a number of fast food chains and restaurants everywhere, offering food at very cheap and affordable rates. These junk foods seem to be very tempting and delicious. We love to spend our money on such worthless and unhealthy food without knowing the consequences and hazards that it will bring to our health. No doubt a fatty burger with a lot of mayonnaise and cheese tastes good but do you actually know that what you are eating? This mouth watering burger you are eating contains a lot of saturated or bad fats and cholesterol, which are responsible for making you obese.

We are living in the era where no one has time for even one's own self. To save our time we prefer ready made and processed foods. Isn't it easy to take out frozen beef steaks from your fridge, frying them and enjoying them just within few minute without taking any pain? Yes it's so but you will have to pay a price in return as well. May be you don't know that how these foods are prepared. The chemical, food additives, preservatives, high sugars, cholesterol and unhealthy fats

contained within these foods are the major for your unwanted weight gain. These unhealthy fats deposit within coronary arteries of heart and increase the risks of heart attacks. This is the price you are paying. If you want to stay fit, lean and healthy then you must be avoiding these foods as much as possible. Always prefer home made foods as they are highly beneficial for health.

Do not eat while watching TV:

Are you eating while sitting in front of TV because you cannot afford to miss your favorite serial? Stop doing this. Because by doing so, your interest will be more towards TV and you will not be able to realize that how much you have eaten. In this way, you're consuming more calories than are being required without even knowing, which forces your body to put on weight

Never skip breakfast:

Skipping your breakfast is the worst way of losing weight. If you're thinking that following a strict diet plan and skipping the meal is going to help you in cutting your belly fat then you're wrong. You must know that having a proper breakfast brings us many health advantages. Skipping the breakfast is not the recommended solution for obesity. If you don't eat breakfast, you will feel more exhausted, weak and deprived of energy. To get your energy back, you would go for day time snacks. These snacks contain high calories which cause weight gain. On the other hand, people who are in habit of taking breakfast remain more energetic and active throughout the day. Such people feel full for longer time and avoid day time snacking.

Herbal remedies for losing weight- "Fall in love with us to get lean and smart" say herbs:

Go green, Go for herbs. Herbs which may help:

- Cinnamon.
- Dandelion.
- Fennel seeds.
- Ginseng.
- Jujube.
- Turmeric.

No one can deny the importance of herbs. Herbal remedies offer you a simple, natural and cost effective solution for obesity. Instead of wasting your money on so called slimming products you can try making your own slimming products and teas at home. The herbs which cause weight loss include:

Cinnamon:

Cinnamon is used as a traditional herb for losing weight. Cinnamon improves the digestion, boosts the metabolism and triggers the calorie burning. Cinnamon also helps in lowering cholesterol level. Cinnamon stabilizes blood sugar level and prevents fat accumulation in body. For making a weight loss drink at home, take a cup of water and add ½ teaspoon of cinnamon powder and 1 teaspoon of honey in it. Drink this honey cinnamon mixture two times a day to get back into shape.

Dandelion:

Dandelion is a very effective and nutritious herb. Dandelion acts on your digestive system, making it able to digest food faster. It stimulates the thyroid gland which leads to weight loss. Dandelion helps in eliminating all harmful toxins and metabolic wastes. Sip the dandelion root tea 1-2 times a day to shed off some extra pounds. You may not like the taste but so many health benefits of this magical herb will encourage you to tolerate its bitter taste.

Fennel seeds:

Fennel seed tea is a guaranteed formula for weight loss. Fennel seeds are known as appetite suppressant. By controlling the hunger, they help in losing weight. Having a cup of fennel seed tea daily stimulates your digestive system to metabolize food more speedily.

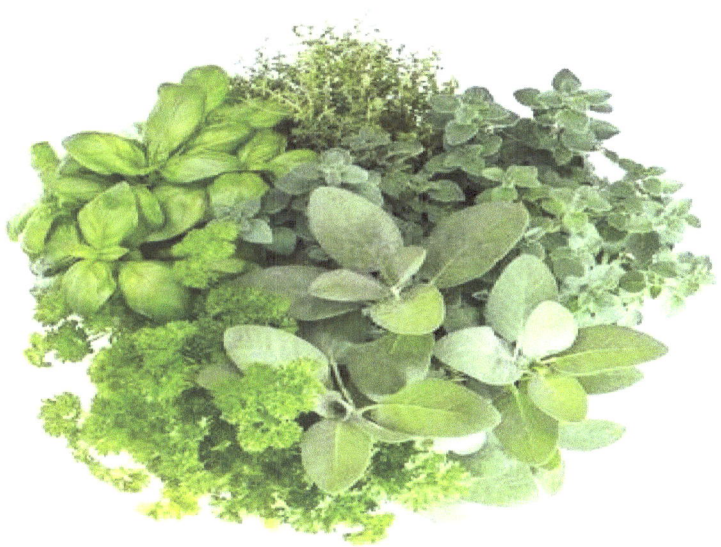

Ginseng:

Ginseng is used as a medicinal herb for treating various ailments. It's regarded as the best treatment for obesity. Ginseng speeds up the

metabolism of carbohydrates, fats and proteins. It amplifies the calorie burning process in your body. The more calories you burn, the more weight you lose. Consuming ginseng root extracts keeps you active, energetic, lean and smart.

Jujube:

Here is another amazing herbal remedy for losing weight. Jujube is a beneficial herb enriched with healthy nutrients like vitamin c, Vitamin B, calcium, phosphorus and iron. Jujube is known for its weight losing effects since ancient time. The antioxidants found within this wonderful herb help in boosting the metabolism. Take a few jujube leaves and soak them in water. Leave it for overnight. Drink this water, containing jujube extracts, in the next morning. Repeating the remedy daily will help you in losing few pounds of weight.

Turmeric:

This yellow orange spice is valued for its potential to cause weight loss. Mix 1 teaspoon of turmeric in a glass of warm water and drink it. Do this daily to lose some weight. Turmeric, like other spices and curries, has the ability to produce heat in body. Obviously when your body gets heated up, it means you are burning extra calories. It's proven through research that turmeric contributes to fat and weight loss by suppressing the formation of fat cells. Turmeric blocks the sprouting of blood vessels needed for the formation of fat cell. Having low number of fat cell means your body won't be able to store any extra fats now.

Exercises for rapid weight loss- "Burn fats, build muscles and get back in shape"

Are you trying to lose weight without doing exercise? Believe me, just relying on the home remedies, herbal solutions and strict diet plan is not enough to see a prominent reduction in weight. You cannot expect a marked reduction in weight without being physically active. Only a healthy physically activity or regular exercise can kick start the rapid weight loss. The more physically active you are, the more energy you need. This leads to fast burning of calories, to meet the energy demands of body. The fat loss workouts include a combination of cardio exercise and heavy weight lifting training.

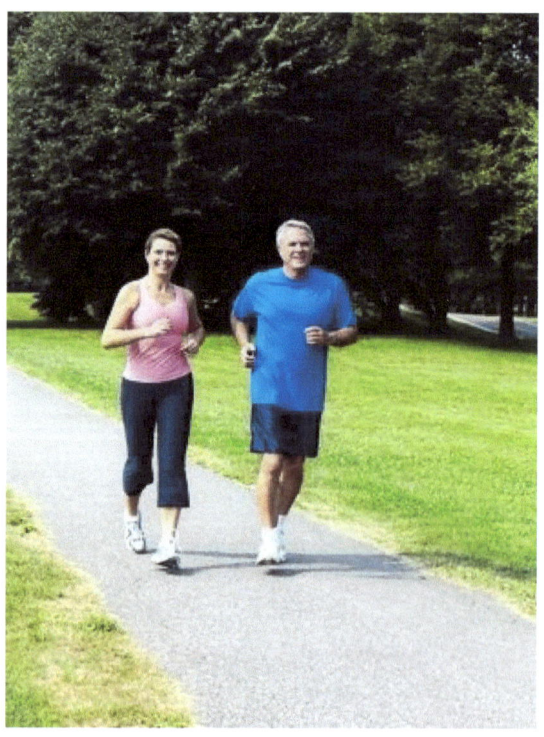

Cardio exercises:

Cardio means "heart". The cardio exercises are those which increase the heart rate. Cardio exercise plan is the best way to lose weight more effectively. Cardio exercises include some low intensity aerobics like running, jogging and swimming etc. The word aerobic is used for these exercises because they increase the oxygen demands of body. While doing the cardio exercise, the metabolic rate of body increases. This in turn raises the oxygen and nutrients requirements of muscles. Oxygen is necessary for carrying out metabolic reactions in muscles and for providing them with energy. To cope up with the oxygen demands of muscle, the heart begins to pump blood at higher rate. The higher the oxygen supply, the higher will be the metabolic rate and calorie burning.

Spend 20-30 minutes daily on cardio workout. Cardio workout helps you in shedding stubborn and undesirable fat. There are varieties of cardio exercises that you can do easily at home. For example doing aerobics will help you burn 800 calories per hour. Similarly, light jogging for 20 minutes burns 300 calories.

Now you fully understand the importance of exercise in maintaining a healthy body weight. In the beginning you might find it difficult to exercise for 30 min. There is no need to over burden you in the start. Stop exercising when you feel completely exhausted and fatigued. This is natural because your body is not used to ir. After a few days your body will adapt and you'll start feeling comfortable with it.

Body weight training and weight lifting:

Weight lifting workouts along with a diet plan helps in losing weight. You might have heard that for weight lifting you'll have to put on some weight first. This is not completely true. The chief purpose of weight lifting is to give your body a perfect and attractive shape. Weight lifting is referred to as building lean muscle mass by cutting down all ugly looking fat. Lifting weights helps in losing weight by increasing the muscle mass. The greater the muscle, the higher will be metabolic rate of body because your bigger muscles need more energy now. In other words, your body needs to burn a large number of calories, which forces you to lose weight.

Doing weight lifting 3 times a week serves multiple purposes at one time. Lifting heavy weights not only reduces weight remarkably but also gives you a desirable and dashing look by giving a tone to your muscles.
If you haven't got access to a gym then you can do body weight exercises like pushups, pull ups ans crunches etc.

Surgical treatment for obesity - "Don't lose hope"

If you've tried all natural remedies to combat your obesity and they failed to bring any visible result, the only option you are left with is the surgical treatment. Surgical treatment is recommended for people having BMI more than 40. Surgery is done only when you lose every hope to get rid of this morbid obesity. Some commonly done surgical procedures are:

Liposuction:

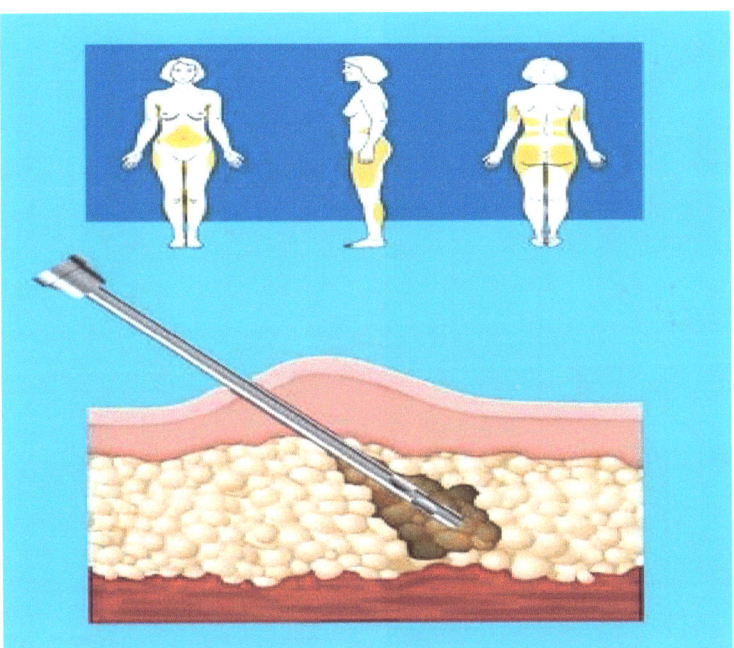

As the name is indicating, the liposuction is the method of fat remodeling with the help of suction or vacuum. The area from where the fats have to be removed is given small incisions. Small suction tubes are inserted through holes into fat tissues and the fats are suctioned through these tubes easily. Ultra sound assisted liposuction is a new technique. In this procedure the ultra sound waves are used to melt the fats which make their suction easier.

Gastric banding:

Gastric banding is the safest and least invasive surgical procedure for treating obesity. Gastric binding is a kind of restrictive surgery which is done to aid weight loss. In gastric banding, a laproscopic method is used to bind a silicone band around the upper part of stomach. Binding the stomach with silicone band creates a small pouch which can hold only a small amount of food. The person who has undergone such surgery won't be able to eat much, which curbs his appetite and promotes weight loss.

Photo Credit
All images licensed by fotolia.com

variety fresh herbs isolated on white

© *LiliGraphie - Fotolia.com*

Diabetes

© *Marco2811 - Fotolia.com*

Herzinfarkt

© *Klaus Eppele - Fotolia.com*

liposuction

© *alexonline - Fotolia.com*

Healthy food

© *Lucian Milasan - Fotolia.com*

Diseased artery with fatty deposits

© *Giovanni Cancemi - Fotolia.com*

Fat Man

© *bicubic - Fotolia.com*

Obesity medical poster design

© *paradox - Fotolia.com*

Seniors couple jogging.

© *Kurhan - Fotolia.com*

homme infarctus

© *dalaprod - Fotolia.com*

Abstract Heart Monitor

© *dvarg - Fotolia.com*

medicine bottle

© *Paulista - Fotolia.com*

Healthy foods in bowl, paleo diet foods, fruits nuts and berries

© neillockhart - Fotolia.com

Author Bio

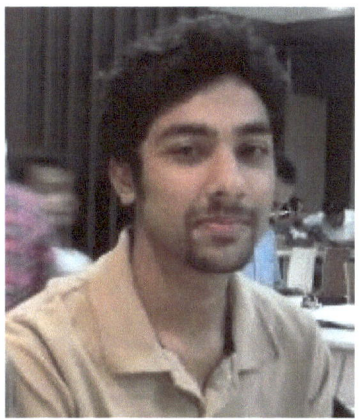

Muhammad Usman is a distinguished medical graduate of Allama iqbal medical college (AIMC). He is a professional writer who has been in the field for more than 4 years. During this time he has produced 10,000+ articles, blogs and eBooks on various niches related to diseases, health, fitness, nutrition and well-being. He is a regular contributor to several journals related to medicine and surgery. He is the editor of several journals and newspapers.

Check out some of the other JD-Biz Publishing books

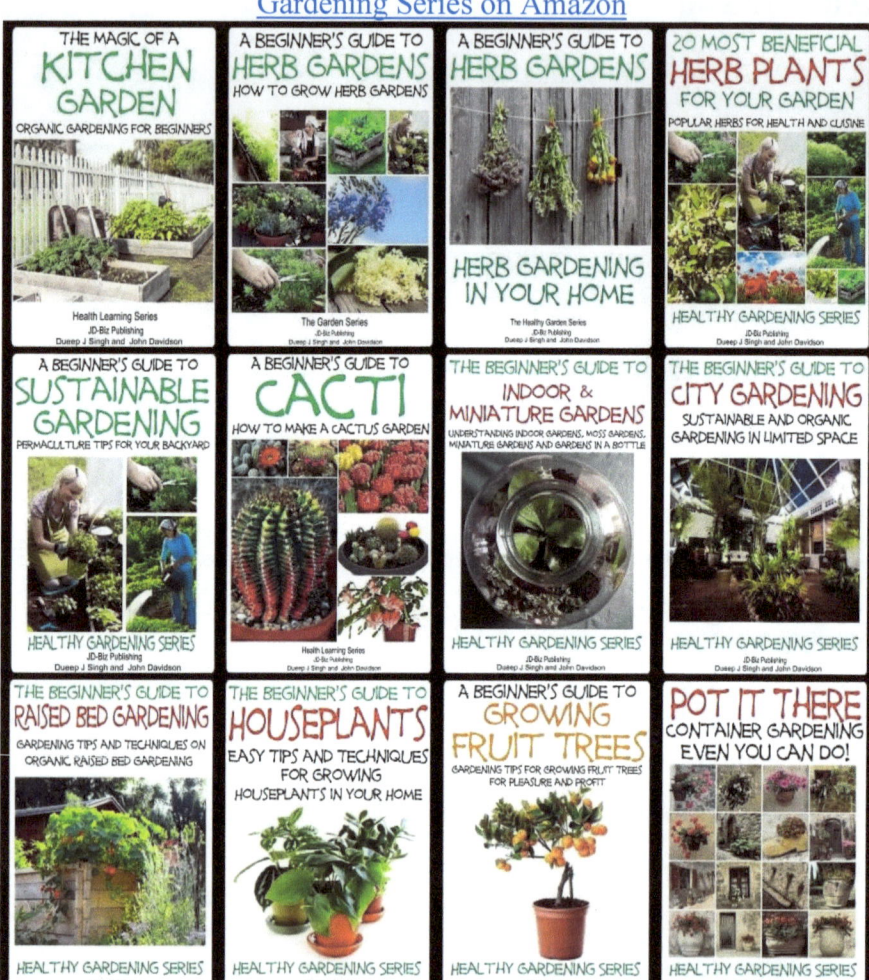

Health Learning Series

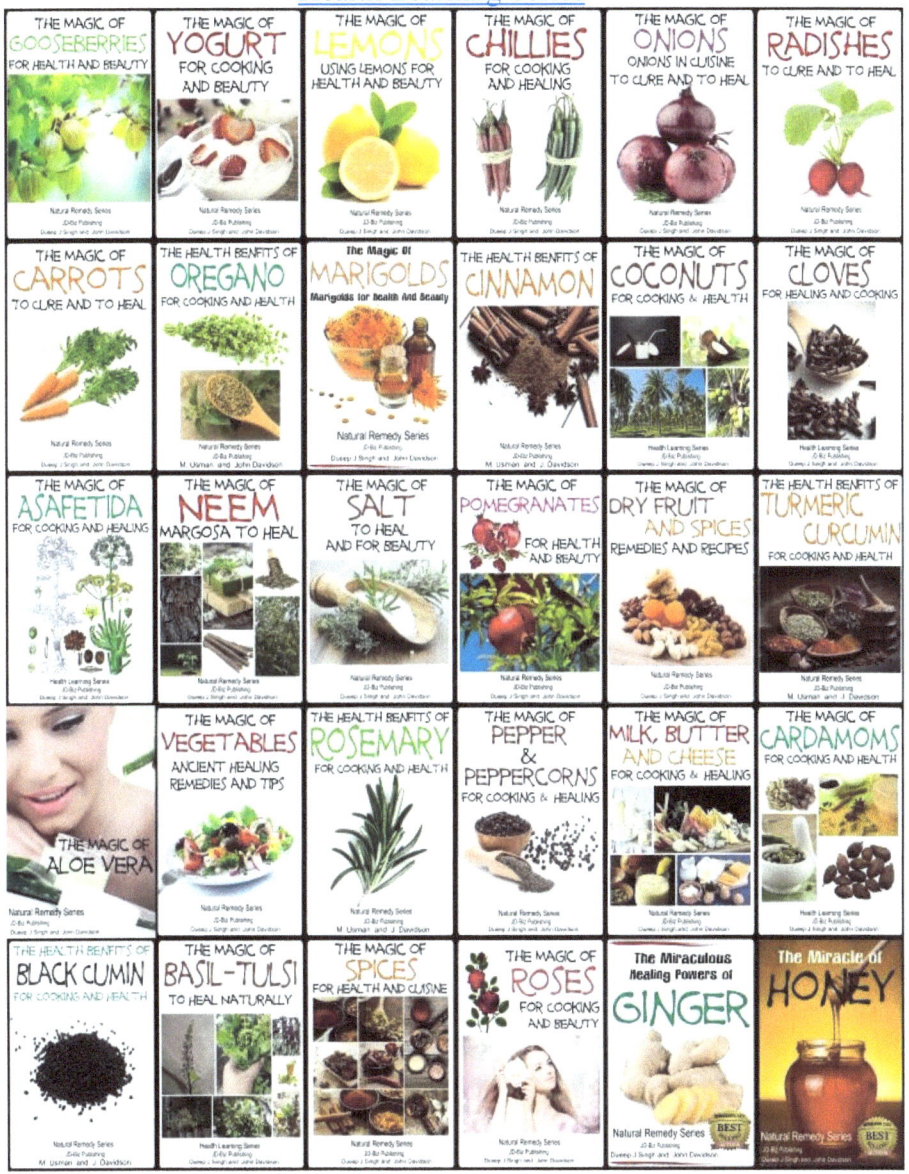

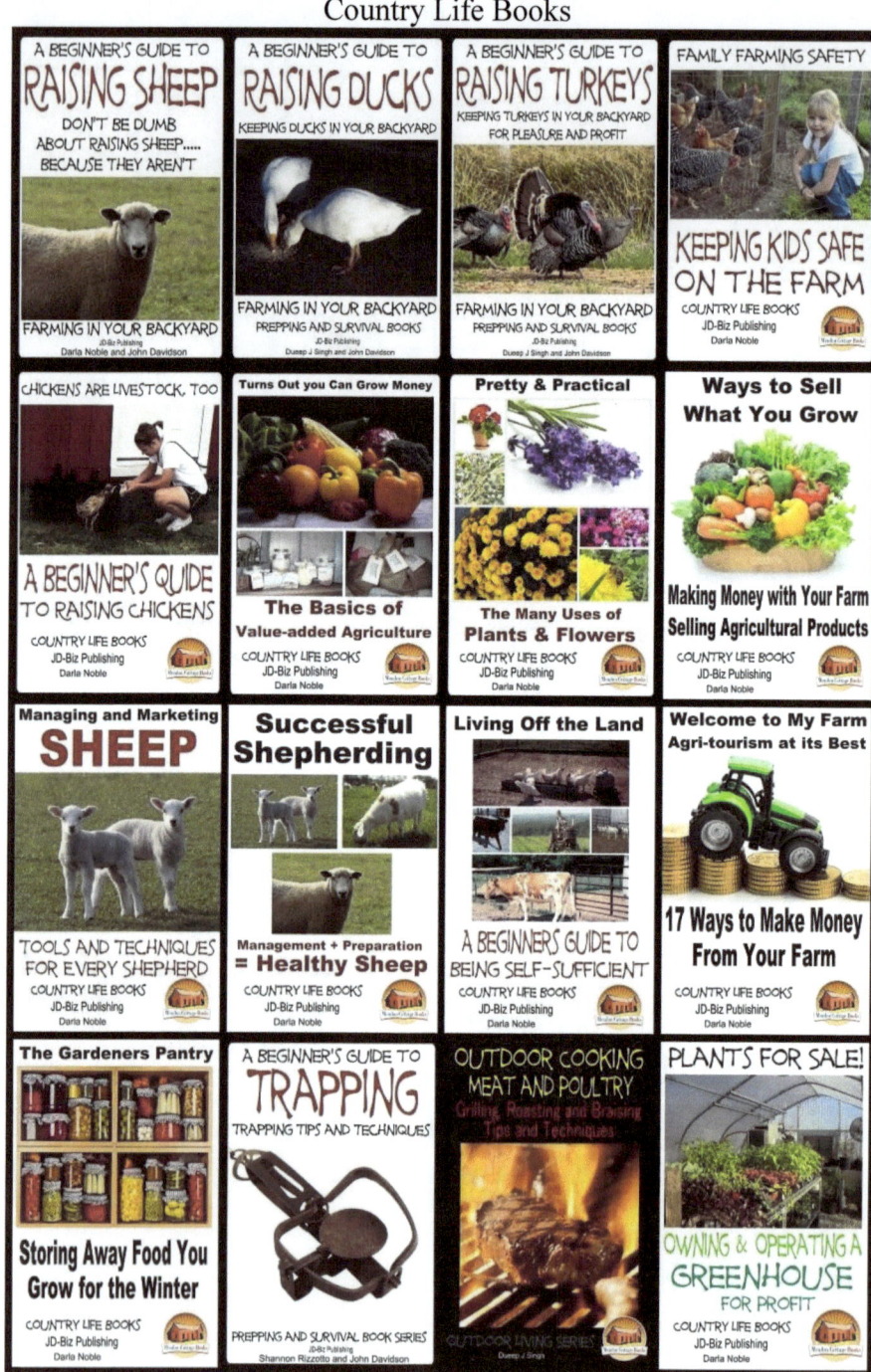

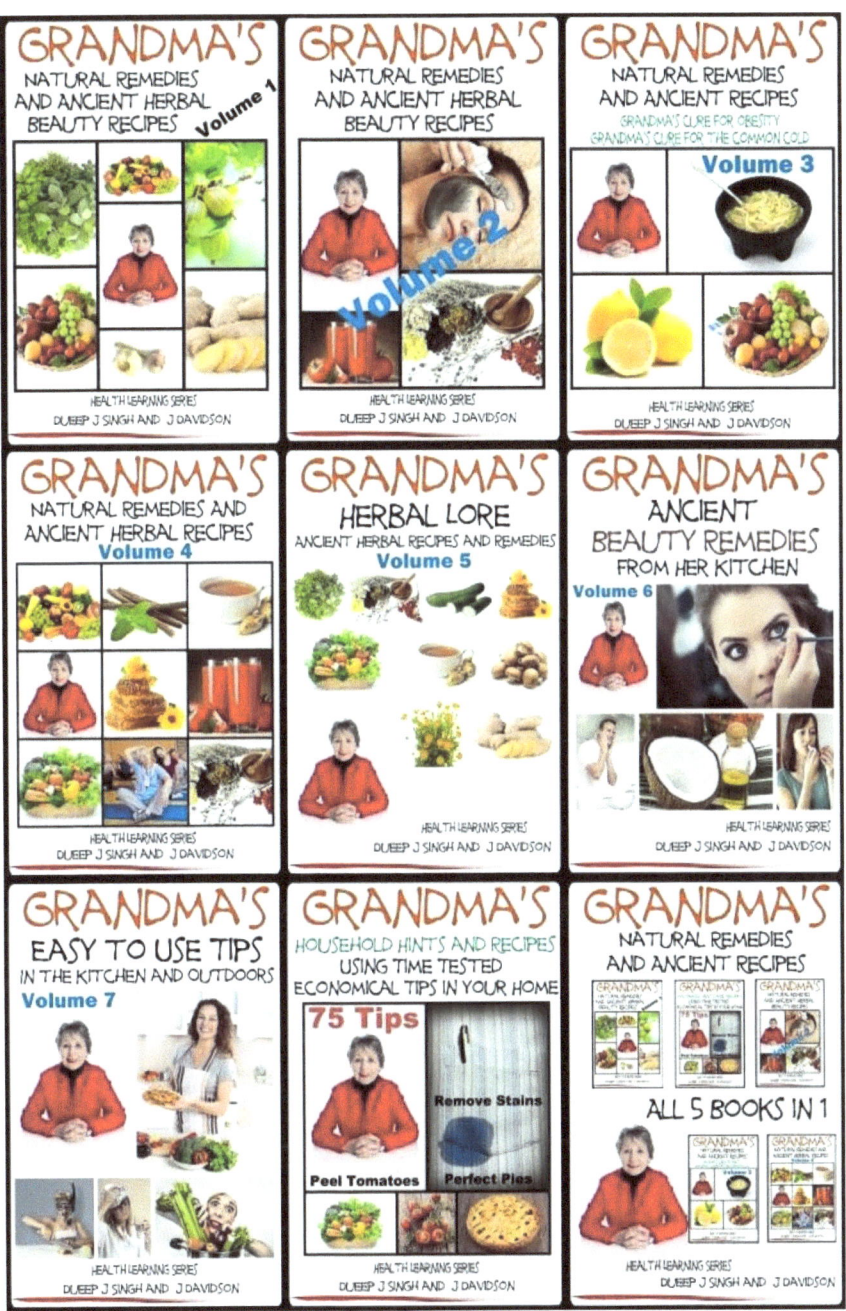

Health Learning Series

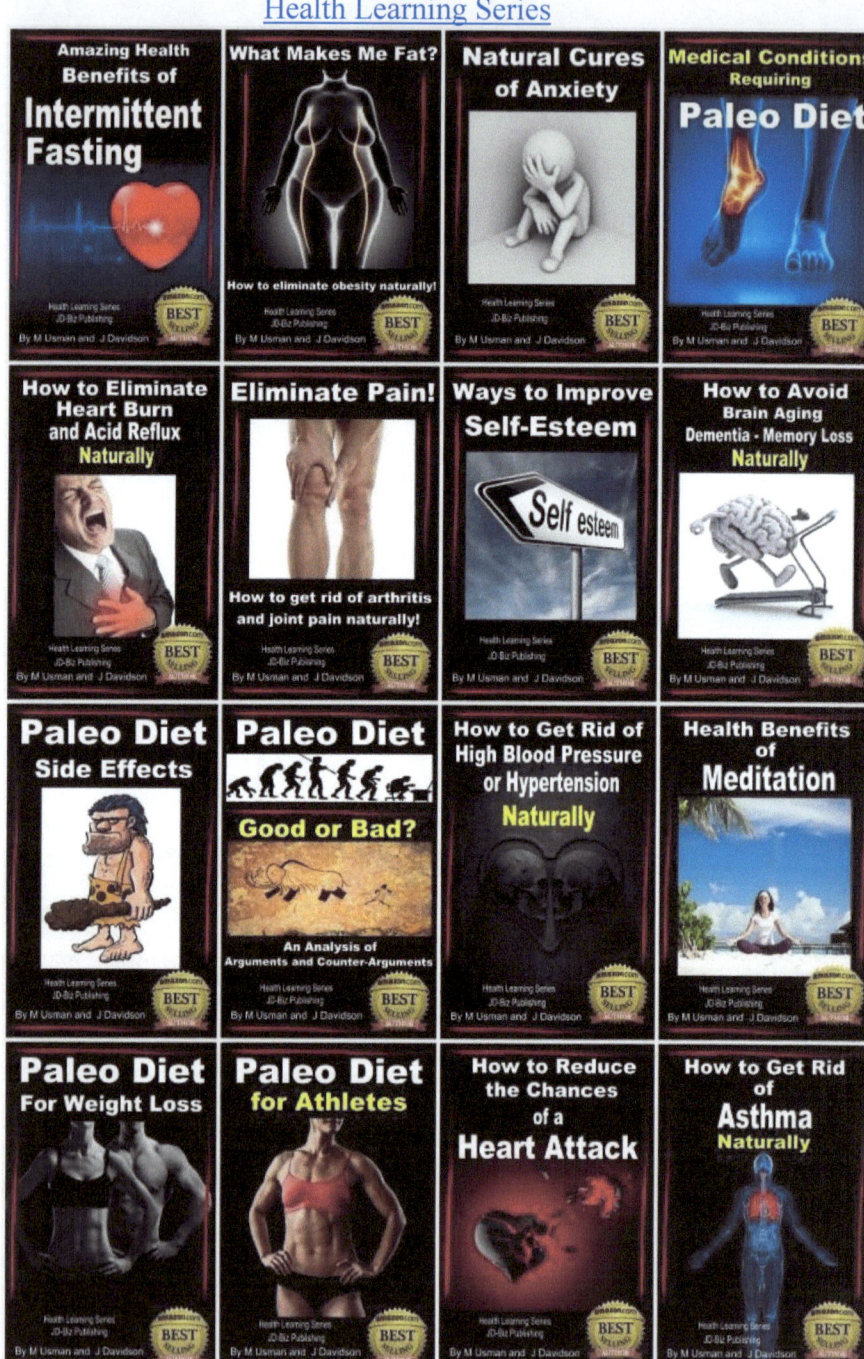

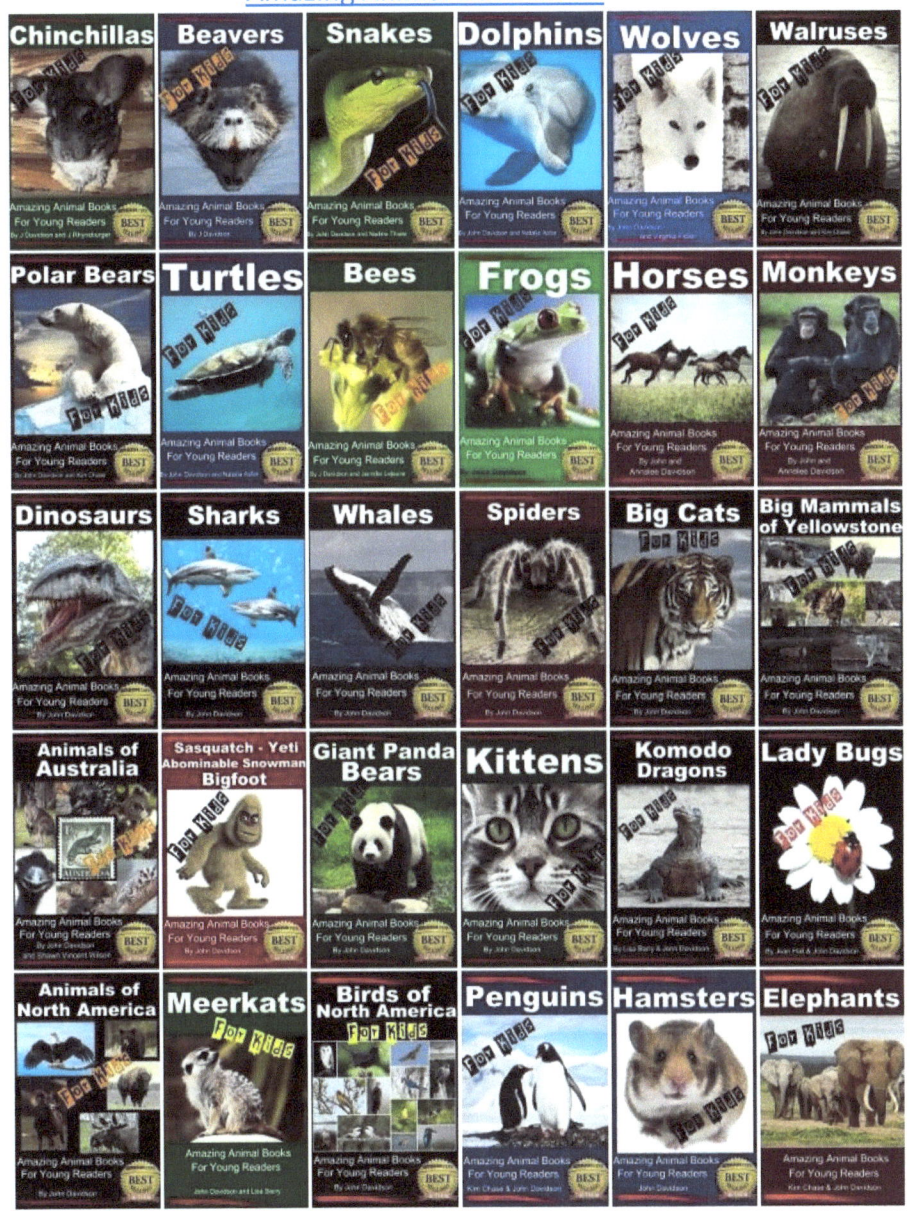

Learn To Draw Series

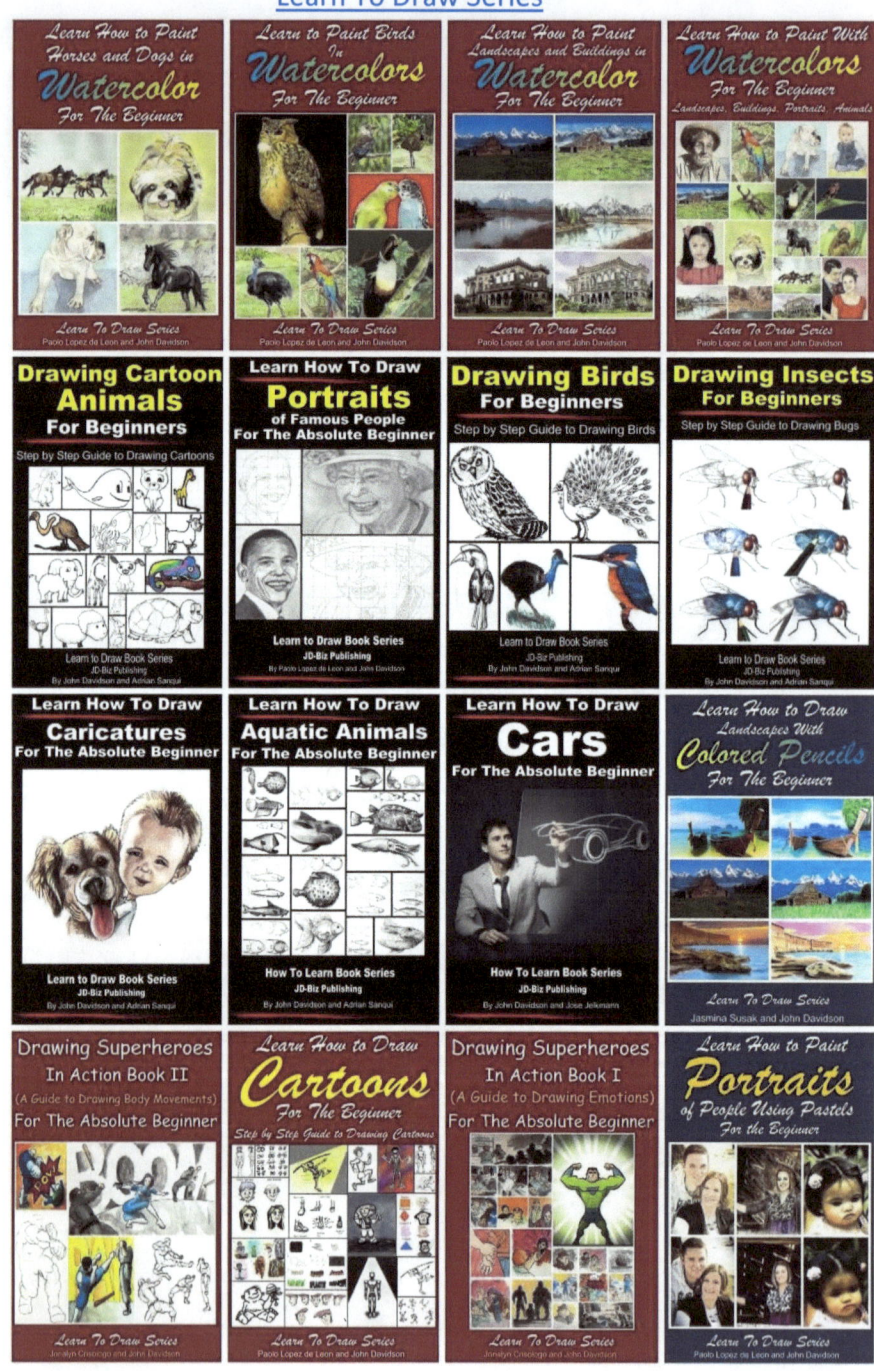

How to Build and Plan Books

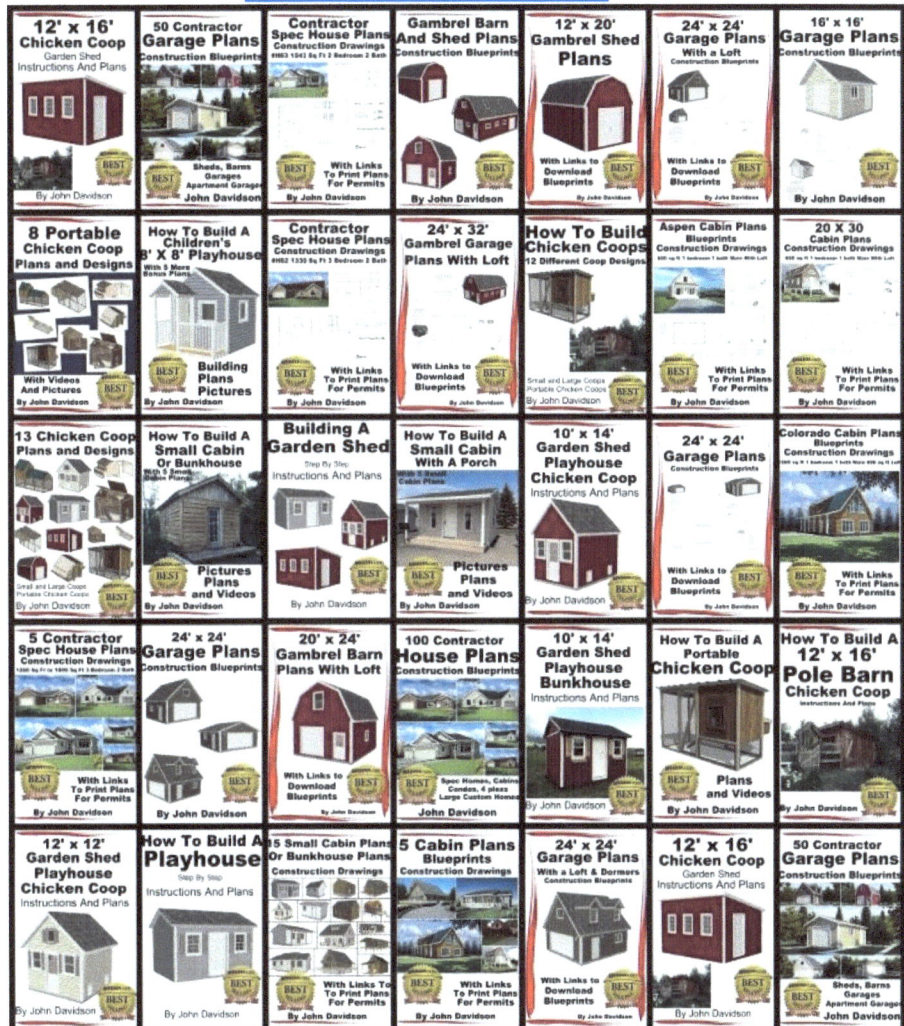

Entrepreneur Book Series

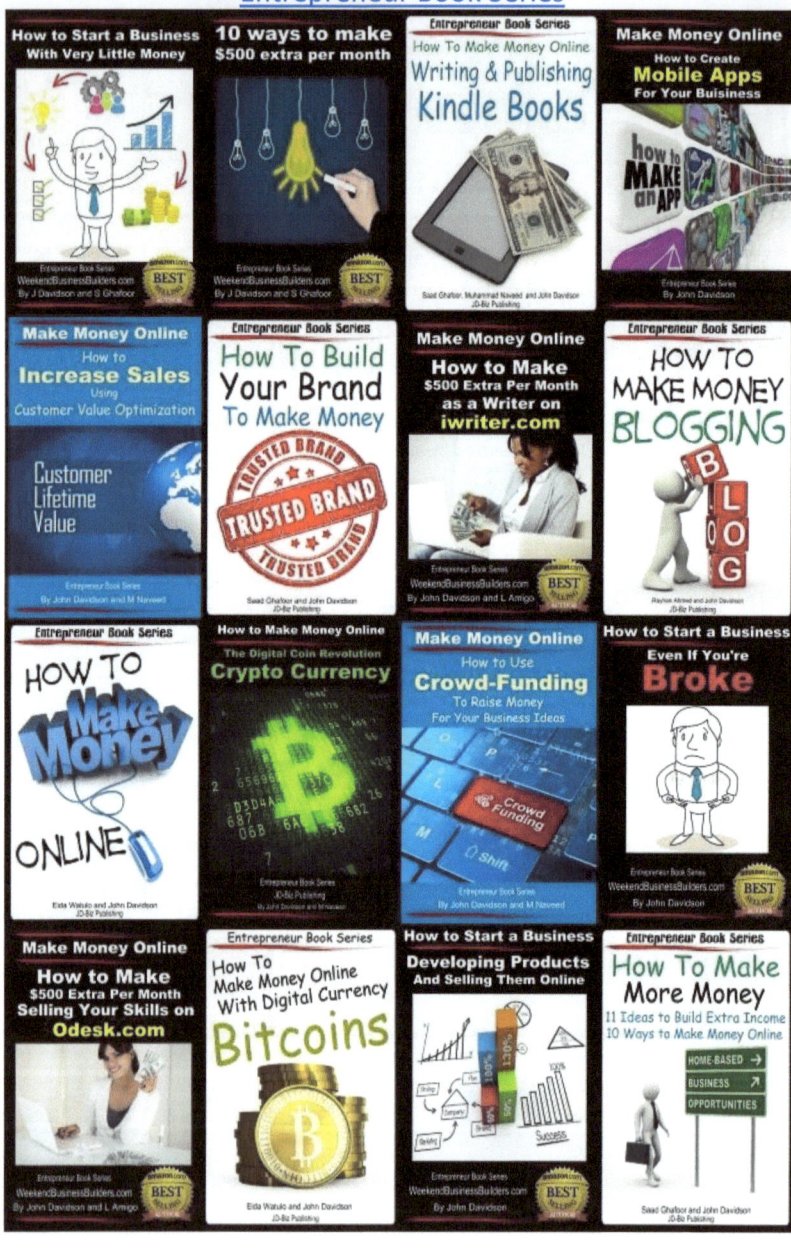

Our books are available at

1. Amazon.com
2. Barnes and Noble
3. Itunes
4. Kobo
5. Smashwords
6. Google Play Books

Download Free Books!
http://MendonCottageBooks.com

Publisher

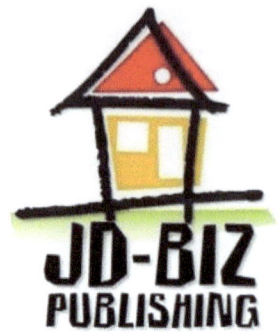

JD-Biz Corp

P O Box 374

Mendon, Utah 84325

http://www.jd-biz.com/

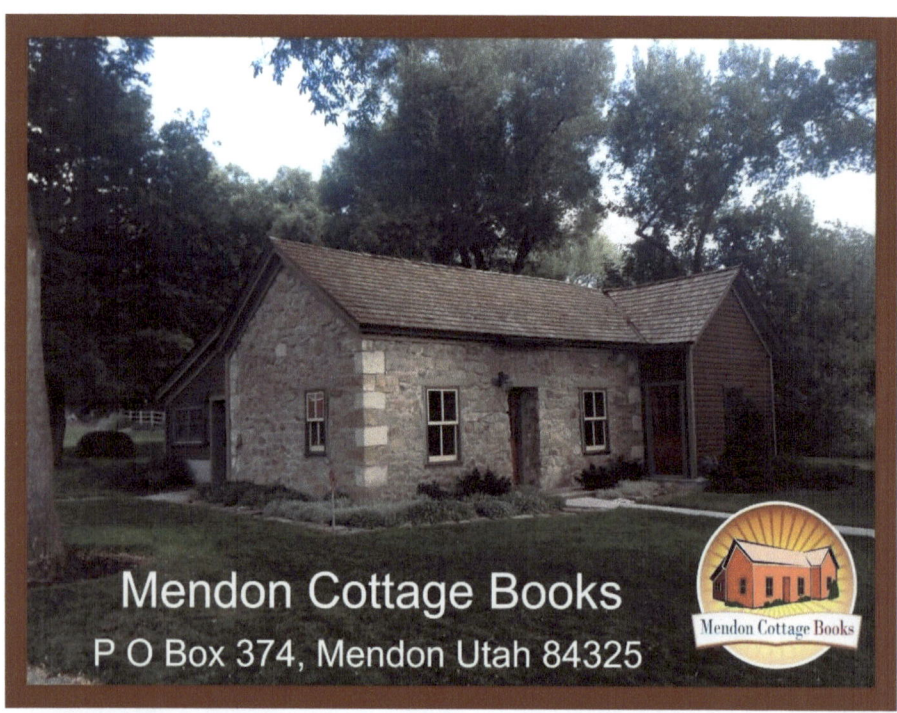

Mendon Cottage Books

P O Box 374, Mendon Utah 84325